Essential Oils for Natural Healing

Discover the Healing Power of These Essential Oils and Live Better… Longer

M.E. Dahkid

ISBN: 1502461838
ISBN-13: 978- 1502461834

DEDICATION

This book is dedicated to those in search of proven methods to improve your health with the help of essential oils.

CONTENTS

INTRODUCTION

Essential oils were mankind's first medicine. From Egyptian hieroglyphics and Chinese manuscripts, we know that priests and physicians have been using essential oils for thousands of years.

Today modern science is rediscovering the wisdom of the ancients. Essential oils are able to reach deep into the recesses of our brains, cross over the chemical barriers, and open the hidden channels within our minds and bodies. Essential oils fragrances pass on to the limbic system of the brain without being registered by the cerebral cortex.

The Benefits of Essential Oils

Essential Oils are regenerating and oxygenating. They are the immune defense properties of plants and are so small in molecular size that they can quickly penetrate the tissues of the skin.

Essential oils are lipid soluble and are capable of penetrating cell walls, even if they have hardened because of an oxygen deficiency. In fact, essential oils can affect every cell of the body within 20 minutes and are then metabolized like other nutrients.

Essential oils contain oxygen molecules which help to transport nutrients to the starving human cells. Because a nutritional deficiency is an oxygen deficiency, disease begins when the cells lack oxygen for proper nutrient assimilation. By providing the needed oxygen, essential oils also work to stimulate the immune system.

Essential oils are very powerful antioxidants. Antioxidants create an unfriendly environment for free radicals. They prevent all mutations, work as free radical scavengers, prevent fungus, and prevent oxidation in the cells.

Essential oils are antibacterial, anti-cancerous, anti-fungal, anti-infectious, anti-microbial, anti- tumorial, anti-parasitic, anti-viral, and antiseptic. Essential oils have been shown to destroy all tested bacteria and viruses while simultaneously restoring balance to the body.

Essential Oil's many Uses

The use of Essential Oils to improve your overall health is called Aromatherapy. The contents of Essential Oils are known as hormones, antibiotics, thermions (unseen scents) and recycling cells (essential to the existence of a live plant) Due to these properties the immunity of plants to various diseases is heightened. Disease causing bacteria and viruses are eliminated.

Essential oils which are normally made from plants contain certain qualities that can benefit our overall health. There are two ways in which essential oils work; psychologically - by way of the body's sense of smell on the central nervous system by vaporizers or smelling of the oils; and physically - through the skin by mixing the oils for massage, foot baths or steam inhalation.

Essential Oils for Natural Healing

CHAPTER 1 – LOVING LAVENDER

The most well-known essential oil, Lavender has anti-bacterial and anti-viral properties which are essential for treating bites, scrapes and stings. It can be used on its own without carrier oil which makes it one of the most accessible oils on the planet. In Latin, Lavender literally means "to wash," so using this essential oil can help you clear off unnecessary toxins in your system and make you feel better about yourself. It is also said that Lavender promotes clarity of mind and improves one's intuition, too.

Properties:

➢ Anti-convulsant

➢ Anti-fungal

➢ Analgesic

> ➤ Antiseptic

> ➤ Anti-inflammatory

Uses and Benefits:

Lavender Oil is useful for:

> ➤ Helping someone sleep better and deal with insomnia;

> ➤ Relieving nervous tension;

> ➤ Healing burns;

> ➤ Aiding against hair loss and helping you grow your hair again;

> ➤ Easing the pain of PMS or Menstrual Problems;

> ➤ Protects you against respiratory infections/problems;

> ➤ Protects you against high blood pressure and heart diseases;

> ➤ Lowers the level of fats and cholesterol in your system;

> ➤ Clears the skin and makes it healthier and more beautiful;

> ➤ Relieving mental stress;

> ➤ And it is also useful in relaxing and calming the mind, as well.

How to Use:

➤ Apply 2 to 4 drops on vital points such as the temples, the nape, and the wrists or on the neck. You may also diffuse it in the room or inhale it directly from the bottle. You can also drop some on a handkerchief or on your blanket shortly before sleeping so that the scent stays with you as you sleep.

Fun Facts:

➤ Research has it that Lavender increases the brain's beta waves. When this happens, relaxation is being promoted, cognition is improved, and depression is lessened.

➤ Talk about Serendipity--The healing properties of Lavender were actually just accidentally discovered by Rene Gatefosse, a French scientist, when he was severely burned while working in a laboratory and accidentally submerged his hand in some Lavender oil. He realized that the oil helped in tissue regeneration and that his wounds have healed without leaving any scars.

How to make Lavender Oil:

➤ Make sure that you use fresh lavender petals and stems. You may plant some lavender so you could harvest what you need in the future.

➤ Clip the flowers into small pieces then bend the

stems so they could easily fit in the jar. Fill up the jar with both the stems and petals but make sure not to stuff it and leave some room to breathe.

➢ Pour some extra virgin olive oil into the jar then put a stopper so there would be no air pockets between the plant and the oil.

➢ Seal the jar and let it sit for around a month. Place it somewhere with direct sunlight then make sure to shake it a bit daily so the oil would be well-mixed.

After a month, remove the stopper then pour the contents into another jar. Make sure that you are able to transfer all of the oil. Throw excess lavender away and store the jar in a cool, dry place.

CHAPTER 2 - SOMETHING'S COMING UP ROSES

Apart from being some of the most beautiful flowers in the world, roses are also good sources essential oils which make them even more beautiful and interesting. Damascus Rose is often used to extract rose essential oil. It's also one of the most fragrant oils out there.

Properties:

➤ Anti-infection

➤ Anti-inflammatory

➤ Anti-hemorrhaging

➤ Scar-reducing

➤ Anti-ulcer

➤ Aphrodisiac

➢ Relaxant

Uses and Benefits:

Rose essential oil is useful because it:

➢ Relieves anxiety;

➢ Stimulates the mind;

➢ Aids against hypertension;

➢ Heals viral infections and bronchitis;

➢ Heals skin conditions such as eczema;

➢ Lessens wrinkles and brings back the moisture of the skin;

➢ Lessens menstrual problems;

➢ Lessens digestive problems;

➢ Aids against liver congestion;

➢ And is also good against headaches, sprains and eye infections.

How to Use:

➢ Apply 2 to 4 drops on vital points. You may also inhale this directly or diffuse it around the room.

Fun Facts:

➢ It is said that most of Cleopatra's cosmetics contained rose in them.

➢ It is also said that rose oil is used to help one's emotions become balanced and is also used in opening the "heart chakra" to let someone be open to new experiences and adventures in life!

How to make Rose Oil:

➢ Fill up a sterilized jar with dry or freshly dried rose petals together with the buds. Break and bruise the petals if you want, as well.

➢ Fill the jar with olive, vegetable or any carrier oil of your choice then put on the lid and shake the jar to make sure that the oil gets distributed evenly.

➢ Place the jar in a cool and dark place for around a month and make sure to shake a bit daily and wipe any excess moisture away.

➢ After a month, have cheesecloth at the ready then squeeze the herbs until they are drained of every drop. What gets left behind in the jar is now considered as your finished oil.

Store in a cool, dry place and use whenever necessary.

M.E. Dahkid

CHAPTER 3 - AMAZING WINTERGREEN

Wintergreen Oil is said to easily associate with each of a person's senses and that's why it can increase the vibrations of the body and promote holistic healing. Back in the day, it was used in religious ceremonies to bring healing and harmony to the earth and its people.

Properties:

➢ Anti-inflammatory

➢ Antiseptic

➢ Analgesic

➢ Anti-spasmodic

➢ Anti-coagulant

➢ Stimulant

➤ Anti-rheumatic

Uses and Benefits:

Wintergreen Oil is beneficial because:

➤ It protects the body against sclerosis;

➤ It alleviates the pain of asthma;

➤ It stimulates the brain;

➤ Alleviates back ache, bone pain and promotes easy healing of fractured bones;

➤ Protects you against cardiovascular conditions;

➤ Protects against Crohn's Disease, Carpal Tunnel Syndrome, Disk Deterioration, Gallstones, Fibromylagia, and different kinds of cramps;

➤ Alleviates the pain of headaches;

➤ Prevents the onset of varicose veins;

➤ It detoxifies the lympathic system;

➤ And protects you against most other diseases such as indigestion, hyperthyroidism, itching, hematoma, hemorrhoids, mumps, kidney stones, Grave's disease, osteoporosis, osteoarthritis and spine injury, as well.

How to Use:

➤ Dilute by a ratio of 20% oil with 80% water then apply 2 to 4 drops on vital points or inhale directly. You may also diffuse this around the room.

Fun Facts:

➢ It is said that Native Americans used to chew Wintergreen so they could have full capacity and endurance in running long distances.

➢ Wintergreen is also said to have a lot to do with helping a person love and accept himself better. It may also lead to introspection and better intuition.

➢ Wintergreen is also usually used as a flavoring for toothpaste, gum and root beer as well.

How to make Wintergreen Oil:

➢ Place torn Wintergreen leaves in a jar until it is about 75% full then pour some extra virgin olive oil in.

➢ Put the lid on and shake the jar to make sure that everything gets mixed together thoroughly. Keep the jar in a dark place for at least a month but make sure to shake the jar every other day.

After 4 to 6 weeks, pour the contents of the jar into another sterilized jar and remove any excess leaves. Store in a cool, dry place and use whenever necessary.

M.E. Dahkid

CHAPTER 4 – GREAT GERANIUM

Geranium Essential Oil comes from over 200 species of Geraniums, the most beneficial of which is the Graveoleons Species that come from Reunion Island in the Indian Ocean. Geranium literally means "stork" in Greek and is said to help diminish the feelings of being abandoned and unloved. It's also part of most first aid kits because of its healing and anti-inflammatory properties.

Properties:

➢ Anti-inflammatory

➢ Anti-bacterial

➢ Anti-fungal

➢ Anti-spasmodic

➢ Diuretic

➢ Sedative

➢ Anti-depressant

➢ Homeostatic (aids in the stoppage of bleeding)

➢ Insect repellant

➢ Pancreas and liver stimulant

➢ Astringent

Uses and Benefits:

Geranium Oil is great because:

➢ It detoxifies the liver and pancreas and rids the body of toxins;

➢ Aids against hepatitis and most diseases of the liver;

➢ Prevents and reduces the risk of fungal infections;

➢ Heals diabetes;

➢ Revitalizes and cleanses the skin and reduces the risk of skin infections such as Psoriasis and Eczema;

➢ Reduces the risk of Herpes;

➢ Protects the body against viral infections;

➢ Balances hormones and prevents menstrual problems;

➢ Helps the mind let go of negative memories and emotions and also eases nervous tension;

➢ And it also aids against insomnia and indigestion.

How to Use:

➢ Dilute with a 50:50 ratio (50% water and 50% oil).

➢ Apply at least 2 to 4 drops to vital points especially to the temples and abdomen for it to be easily absorbed.

➢ You may also diffuse this around the house/room or inhale it directly.

Fun Facts:

➢ The first Geranium Oil was made by the French Chemist Recluz in 1819 by distilling the leaves of the said plant.

➢ In the 1600s, European Gardeners and Farmers used to plant Geranium to ward off Evil Spirits!

➢ It is also called Geranium because its fruit looks like the bill of a stork.

➢ Geranium Oil is also sometimes used as a calming body scrub to refresh and calm the body.

How to make Geranium Oil:

➢ Cut some Rose Geranium flowers, stems and leaves that are enough to fill up a jar up to 1/3 inch towards the top. Make sure that you place a lot of leaves in because they contain the highest amount of oil.

➢ Use a wooden spoon to stir leaves, flowers and

stems together and make sure that oils are released. Don't mash them up so be careful with stirring then press them lightly to the bottom of the jar.

➢ Pour olive or jojoba oil in the jar then cover the jar and shake so everything will be well-blended. Place the jar outside for around 48 hours then swirl once every few hours.

Pour the contents to the cheesecloth and use it as a sieve to remove excess leaves, flowers and stems then pour the contents into another jar and store. Use as needed.

CHAPTER 5 – SLEEP WELL WITH SANDALWOOD

Coming from the heart of evergreen trees in Southeast Asia, Sandalwood Oil is known as a sleeping agent. If you're suffering from insomnia, then this will surely help you sleep well again. It is also said to be ultimately relaxing and is best used during bedtime to help you sleep easily and get you ready for the following day.

Properties:

➢ Anti-viral

➢ Anti-depressant

➢ Anti-tumors

➢ Aphrodisiac

➢ Antiseptic

➢ Astringent

➢ Bronchial dilator

➢ Immune system stimulant

➢ Tonic

➢ Sedative

Uses and Benefits:

You should try Sandalwood Oil because:

➢ It regenerates cells, takes care of the hair and skin, and prevents the onset of acne and most skin conditions;

➢ Aids in better sleeping patterns and reduces the risk of insomnia;

➢ Prevents impotency;

➢ Relaxes and calms both the mind and body;

➢ Prevents and reduces the risk of hemorrhoids;

➢ Protects the body against viral infections such as bronchitis as well as common coughs, colds and flu;

➢ Protects the body against diarrhea;

➢ And it also protects the body against most cancers and ulcers.

How to Use:

➢ Apply around 2 to 4 drops on the wrists, ankles

and other vital points.

➤ Inhale directly or diffuse it around the room shortly before sleeping.

Fun Facts:

➤ Back in the olden times, Sandalwood was used to help in embalming the dead and making sure that their souls were released during their funerals. Interesting!

➤ In 78 AD, a book entitled "Dioscorides in de Materia Medica" was filled up with descriptions of different plants and Sandalwood was considered as a healing plant. That's why since then until the 17th century, Sandalwood was considered as a medicine.

➤ Because of the aromatic and sweet scent of wood, Sandalwood naturally relaxes the mind deeply.

How to make Sandalwood Oil:

➤ Pre-heat oven to 200 degrees then pour a cup of the carrier oil in the saucepan and add the sandalwood powder. Stir until well-combined.

➤ Cover the saucepan then put it in the oven and cook the oil and sandalwood together for around 2 to 4 hours. Make sure to stir frequently to prevent it from getting burned.

➤ Use cheesecloth to strain the mixture then pour contents into another jar. Use whenever necessary.

M.E. Dahkid

CHAPTER 6 – ROMAN CHAMOMILE GOODNESS

It is said that Roman Chamomile Oil promotes inner peace and may help remind someone of days gone by because of its "nostalgic" and sweet scent. Roman Chamomile is also one of the most popular and beneficial essential oils around as it is truly calming and relaxing and promotes holistic healing. Literally, Chamomile means "Greek Apple" which is said to resonate one's childhood and innocence, also making it one of the best essential oils for babies. The topmost flowers are used to create the essential oil.

Properties:

➢ Anti-spasmodic

➢ Nerve regenerative

➢ Anti-inflammatory

➢ Anti-parasitic

➢ Relaxant

➢ Detoxifying

Uses and Benefits:

Roman Chamomile Oil is worth trying because:

➢ It aids against anxiety, depression and insomnia;

➢ It protects the skin against infections and also regenerates cells and tissues to make you healthy and younger looking;

➢ It tranquilizes the nervous system;

➢ It detoxifies the liver;

➢ Relieves menstrual problems and PMS;

➢ And it also protects the body against digestive problems and Attention Deficit Hyperactivity Disorder (ADHD), as well.

How to Use:

➢ Apply 2 to 4 drops to ankles, wrists and other vital points.

➢ You may also have it diffused or inhale it directly.

➢ You may also use Roman Chamomile Oil by pouring 2 to 3 drops of it in your bath water.

Fun Facts:

➢ Roman Chamomile was dedicated to the sun god Ra in Ancient Egypt.

➢ It is also said that Roman Chamomile helps someone accept himself for who he really is and opens up the heart and mind to make one ready for whatever life throws at him and become more thankful for what he has in life.

➢ Back then, Roman Chamomile was also mixed with flour as a remedy for spleen, stomach and liver problems and was used by mothers to protect their children against toothaches and stomachaches, too!

How to make Roman Chamomile Oil:

➢ Buy some dead chamomile flowers. Or, you may also choose to grow your own chamomiles then pick them up and clean them. Discard any debris or sand/soil.

➢ Place the flowers on a cutting board to dry them completely.

➢ Next, take a glass jar and have it sterilized then pour some olive oil into the jar up to at least ½ inch near the top.

➢ Add chamomile flowers then stir until each flower is covered and make sure that the flowers have been submerged in oil totally. Put the lid on tightly.

➢ Put the jar in an area under direct sunlight then leave it be for around 2 weeks or until flowers are spent.

➢ Transfer the oil into another clean jar then sieve out any flowers left behind. Strain until no more

flowers are left.
Stir well and store in a cool, dry place.

CHAPTER 7 – JAZZY JASMINE

Jasmine Oil is extracted solely from the flowers of the said plant and is also known as "Queen of the Night" because it is best used before sleeping and the flowers are naturally more aromatic at night and is mainly used to bring happiness. Literally, the name "Jasmine" means "Young Girl". It is also known for its healing properties and the fact that it takes care of the reproductive system more than any other oil does.

Properties:

- ➤ Anti-depressant

- ➤ Anti-bacterial

- ➤ Anti-catarrhal

Uses and Benefits:

Jasmine Oil is amazing because:

- ➤ It aids against anxiety, depression and insomnia;

- ➤ Prevents respiratory problems and hepatitis;

> ➤ Clears and rejuvenates the skin and protects it against most infections and diseases;

> ➤ Promotes hormonal balance and reduces the risk of menstrual problems and PMS;

> ➤ Relaxes and uplifts the mind;

> ➤ Prevents uterine and reproductive disorders;

> ➤ And, it also protects the body against dysentery, muscle spasms and sexually-related problems.

How to Use:

> ➤ Use it undiluted then apply 2 to 4 drops on vital points.

> ➤ Inhale directly or diffuse it around the room.

Fun Facts:

> ➤ Another term for Jasmine is "Moonlight of the Grove."

> ➤ It is also said that using Jasmine Oil helps a person let go of his/her fears and awakens his sexual prowess and makes him understand the importance of true love and intimacy. Jasmine was even used as an aphrodisiac during the time of the Roman Empire!

> ➤ In Japan, some leaders diffuse Jasmine in the office to promote mental clarity and alertness, believing that it makes workers more productive.

How to make Jasmine Oil:

➢ Place jojoba or extra virgin olive oil together with Jasmine Petals in a jar then put the lid on and shake the mixture thoroughly.

➢ Open the jar then pull or bruise the petals then shake again.

➢ Place the jar in a sunny place for around 48 hours and make sure to shake the jar every 12 hours then remove the lid and pour the mixture into another jar. Use muslin cloth as a sieve then pour the mixture back in the jar and leave outside for another 48 hours.

➢ Keep the jar in a cool, dry place and use whenever necessary.

M.E. Dahkid

CHAPTER 8 – TREAT OF TANGERINE

Tangerine Essential Oil is made out of Tangerine Rind. It is often used as a sedative because of its great calming properties. This oil is also a good source of Vitamin C, which makes it an amazing anti-inflammatory agent. It also contains high amounts of Potassium and Magnesium.

Properties:

➢ Anti-coagulant

➢ Anti-tumors

➢ Sedative

➢ Laxative

➢ Detoxifying

➢ Circulatory enhancer

➢ Digestive aid

➢ Anti-spasmodic

➢ Anti-inflammatory

➢ Decongestant

Uses and Benefits:

Tangerine Oil is truly amazing because it:

➢ Prevents and lessens the formation of cellulites;

➢ Prevents poor blood circulation and protects the body against cardio-vascular diseases;

➢ Aids against insomnia and poor digestion;

➢ Protects the liver against hepatitis and most diseases;

➢ Prevents the production and infestation of parasites;

➢ Prevents swelling and obesity;

➢ And it also helps the body absorb water easily, making sure that you are hydrated all the time.

How to Use:

➢ Dilute with 50% water then apply 2 to 4 drops on vital points.

➢ You may also use this with a diffuser or just inhale it directly.

Fun Facts:

➤ Tangerines have been one of China's essential plants for over 3,000 years now!

➤ Tangerine is also high in Folate which makes it great for pregnant and lactating women.

How to make Tangerine Oil:

➤ Scrape off the peel of the tangerine. It would be helpful to use a citrus zester.

➤ Next, fill a glass bottle or jar with the tangerine zest then mix some olive oil inside the jar. Make sure that the tangerine is completely covered in oil.

➤ Put the jar somewhere sunny and just leave it be for 2 to 4 weeks but make sure to shake it every one or two days.

➤ Strain the mixture and discard any excess tangerine peels. Store in a cool, dry place and use as needed.

CHAPTER 9 – TERRIFIC TEA TREE

If you hate mosquitoes and any other insects literally bugging you, then Tea Tree Oil is your friend. It protects you against insect bites by repelling insects away plus it is also known to strengthen the immune system, making it one of the best essential oils out there. It is also said that tea tree oil helps a weak person feel stronger and prevents one from wallowing in self-pity.

Properties:

➢ Anti-bacterial

➢ Anti-viral

➢ Anti-inflammatory

➢ Decongestant

➢ Anti-fungal

➢ Anti-septic

➢ Anti-oxidant

➢ Anti-parasitic

➢ Immune system stimulant

➢ Tissue/cell regenerator

➢ Insect repellant

Uses and Benefits:

You should use Tea Tree Oil because:

➢ It protects you against most fungal infections such as lung viruses, sinus and ringworm;

➢ It protects against bronchitis, tonsillitis, colds and flu;

➢ It clears the hair of dandruff;

➢ It protects you against most skin conditions such as scars and acne;

➢ It helps the body absorb water easily;

➢ It protects you against Candida or Yeast Infections;

➢ It cleanses and refreshes the mind and the body;

➢ And it also prevents other diseases such as hypertension, gum diseases and heart problems, as well.

How to Use:

➤ Dilute with one part essential oil and one part vegetable oil.

➤ Apply 2 to 4 drops on vital points.

➤ You may also use this via a diffuser or by inhalation.

Fun Facts:

➤ Captain James Cook, the famous British Explorer, actually coined the name "Tea Tree" after finding some dark leaves that could create a spicy kind of tea. From that day on, the tea was used both as a drink and a remedy by other British explorers, as well.

➤ Tea Tree Oil is also sometimes called "snake oil" because it detoxifies the effect of a snake bite. That's why you have to have it with you if you're going out in the wild!

➤ In 1933, the British Medical Journal stated that Tea Tree Oil is a very powerful disinfectant and it is non-irritating and non-poisonous which means that it is very safe to use. It is also said to be 12 times stronger than most medicines such as Carbolic Acid.

How to make Tea Tree Oil:

➤ Put some tea tree leaves in a pot and cover it with water then place a measuring cup in a vegetable steamer.

➢ Boil the leaves on high heat and steam half of it in the vegetable steamer then put 4 ice cubes to hasten condensation.

➢ Turn off the burner once all the ice has melted then take off the lid and pour ice down the sink.

➢ Pour the contents of the measuring cup into a jar. Use a funnel to make sure that nothing gets discarded.

➢ Invert the funnel so pressure could be released and then wait for the oil to float above the water. Put the glass in the stockpot and drain the water. Repeat process with the remaining leaves.

Place contents in a jar and store in a cool, dry place. Use whenever necessary.

CHAPTER 10 – LIVING WITH LEMONS

Lemon Essential Oil contains more vitamins than most fruits and vegetables and that's why it's very important that you make it a part of your life. It's also very beneficial in taking care of the hair, scalp, respiratory and digestive system. It is said that Lemons were first planted in Asia and so they were once called as "Median Apples".

Properties:

> Anti-fungal

> Anti-tumors

> Immune system stimulant

> Diuretic

> Anti-viral

> Anti-bacterial

➢ Calming

➢ Expectorant

➢ Astringent

Uses and Benefits:

Lemon is not just a delicious fruit. When made into an essential oil, it's amazing because:

➢ It rejuvenates the skin and helps it remain healthy and young-looking and protects the skin against most infections and diseases such as acne and Psoriasis;

➢ Prevents the memory from being impaired and makes sure that you remain smart and that your mind is on tip-top shape all the time;

➢ Protects the hair from dandruff and from breaking apart;

➢ It protects you against diseases such as gout and urinary tract infections;

➢ It cleanses and detoxifies the liver and the kidney;

➢ Prevents the body from being infested by parasites;

➢ Prevents the onset of varicose veins;

➢ And it also prevents anxiety and insomnia.

How to Use:

➤ Dilute with 50% oil and 50% water.

➤ Apply around 2 to 4 drops on the body's vital points or inhale directly.

➤ You may also diffuse this around the room/house.

Fun Facts:

➤ Early Romans used lemon rind in order to wash clothes and repel insects.

➤ It is also said that Lemon is a symbol of youth and beauty.

➤ Lemon is also said to cleanse the mind and spirit and helps someone become joyful all the time.

➤ In Japanese offices, some supervisors who diffused lemon oil in their workplace saw that the workers became more efficient and mistakes were reduced by at least 54 percent! And that's why it is said that lemon is effective in ensuring mental accuracy.

How to make Lemon Oil:

➤ Grate the lemon outside a bowl.

➤ Next, fill up a glass bottle with the grated lemon zest then add some olive oil in the bottle.

➤ Place the bottle in a sunny place, preferably a windowsill then leave it for around 2 weeks and make sure to stir occasionally.

➤ After 2 weeks, pour the oil in another clean glass bottle and keep it covered. Store and use as needed.

CHAPTER 11 – CLARITY WITH CLARY SAGE

Clary Sage Oil is said to be a woman's best friend because it alleviates the pain from most reproductive diseases, produces hormones and is also rich in anti-oxidants, which means that one's hair, skin and body will be well-protected through the regeneration of cells and tissues. Clary Sage actually literally means "to heal" or "to clear".

Properties:

- Anti-oxidant

- Anti-coagulant

- Anti-tumors

- Sedative

- Astringent

- Anti-cholesterol

- ➢ Anti-diabetic

- ➢ Nerve tonic

Uses and Benefits:

Clary Sage can help make you feel better because:

- ➢ It prevents and alleviates PMS and Menstrual Problems and also prevents hormonal imbalance;

- ➢ Prevents pre-menopausal problems;

- ➢ It prevents impotence;

- ➢ It prevents insomnia and reduces the risk of anxiety and depression;

- ➢ It protects you against viral problems such as bronchitis.

- ➢ It can calm the mind and prevent panic or anxiety attacks from happening and makes you ready for whatever you have to do. It quiets the mind because it is spicy and euphoric;

- ➢ And it also protects you against liver and kidney problems.

How to Use:

- ➢ Dilute with equal parts of water and oil.

- ➢ Apply at least 2 to 4 drops on vital points.

- ➢ Inhale directly or diffuse it around the room.

Fun Facts:

➤ In the middle ages, Clary Sage was also called "Clear Eyes" because once you make an infusion out of the seeds, it can treat eye infections!

➤ Clary Sage is actually part of the Mint family so it's also known for its cooling effect.

➤ In Oriental Medicine, Clary Sage is essential for the proper circulation of blood and for strengthening stuck energies in the body to make sure that the body is well-sustained through all time.

How to make Clary Sage Oil:

➤ Place some Clary Sage in a large glass bottle and crush the leaves to make sure that the jar is stuffed. Fill up the glass up to its neck.

➤ Pour warm carrier oil (such as jojoba, vegetable or extra virgin olive oil) into the bottle then cover it and shake it lightly.

➤ Keep the bottle in a warm and dark place for around 3 days and make sure to stir every 12 hours.

➤ Take out the bottle after 3 days and strain the contents through cheesecloth.

Pour contents into another bottle and use whenever necessary.

M.E. Dahkid

CHAPTER 12 – GRATEFUL FOR GRAPEFRUIT

While not the most popular of essential oils, Grapefruit Oil is actually very beneficial because it prevents the onset of skin, pancreatic, and liver cancer and is quite mentally uplifting as it can prevent depression and anxiety. Plus, Grapefruit Oil also prevents the onset of Breast Cancer by at least 80 percent! Wow!

Properties:

➢ Anti-septic

➢ Anti-tumors

➢ Metabolic stimulant

➢ Fat dissolving

➢ Diuretic

➢ Detoxifying

➢ Tonic

➢ Disinfectant

Uses and Benefits:

Grapefruit Oil is quite important because:

➢ It prevents digestive problems such as dyspepsia and promotes healthy and proper digestion;

➢ It prevents anxiety and Alzheimer's Disease;

➢ It protects the body against cellulites and protects the hair from dandruff and breakage;

➢ It alleviates the risk of liver diseases;

➢ It cleanses the lymph nodes and kidneys;

➢ Its aroma is very refreshing to the mind;

➢ It helps one clear his mind and let go of his worries and frustrations and is said to help someone find his purpose;

➢ And, it also prevents obesity and helps the body's metabolic rates go higher and also helps the body absorb water easily.

How to Use:

➢ Dilute with 50% oil and 50% water then apply around 2 to 4 drops on vital points.

➢ Inhale directly or diffuse around the room.

Fun Facts:

➢ The Grapefruit is actually a hybrid between an orange and a pomelo—which means that you're getting a lot of Vitamin C because these fruits have high contents of that.

➢ It was in the 18th century when Captain Shaddock, an Englishman, cultivated the first couple of Grapefruits in the world. Grapefruits were first called "shaddocks" but were eventually called "Grapefruit" because they look like Grapes.

➢ In Barbados, Grapefruits were considered forbidden fruits but are now regarded among the country's seven wonders! Awesome!

➢ In 1823, Count Odette Philippe brought the Grapefruit to the United States via the Tampa Harbor.

How to make Grapefruit Oil:

➢ Make sure to choose grapefruits with thick rinds because they are the best ones to use in essential oils. Wash the fruit thoroughly then peel it and scrape the pith out before discarding it. It would also be good to use a kitchen grater for this. Collect the rind.

➢ Spread the rind in a plate then let it dry in an area with proper ventilation.

➢ Fill a jar with grapefruit rind then add almond oil up to the top of the jar then cover the jar and let it sit somewhere sunny. Leave it there for 2 weeks.

➢ After 2 weeks, pour the oil in a bowl layered with cheesecloth and discard any excess fruit residue.

Squeeze the rinds to produce more oil.

➢ Pour the oil into glass bottles then seal and store. Use whenever necessary and make sure not to refrigerate.

Please Leave a Review

Finally, if you enjoyed this book, please take the time to share your thoughts and post a review on Amazon. It'd be greatly appreciated!

That review and feedback will help me improve the content in my books – and make each and every one more relevant and helpful to you.

Thank you again and good luck!

M.E. Dahkid